Mushroom Nutrition and Mushroom Supplements: The Bottom line on Mushroom Health Benefits

Agaricus Blazei, Agarikon, Black Trumpet, Turkey Tail, Cordyceps, Lion's Mane, Maitake, Oyster Mushroom, Poria cocos, Reishi, Shiitake Mushrooms

By Mackenzie Logan

Mushroom Nutrition and Mushroom Supplements: The Bottom line on Mushroom Health Benefits

This book is not intended as a substitute for the medical advice of a physician. The reader should regularly consult a physician in matters relating to his/her health and particularly with respect to any symptoms that may require diagnosis or medical attention. No copyright on images, sources attributed where applicable.

"Nutritional mushrooms are one of the most promising and highest performing nutrition and 'curative' natural food source found to date. The challenge is, 'what mushrooms for what ailment'? That's the purpose of this direct, to the point, no fluff volume. This book was written for those interested in information on the following mushrooms, what they can do for you, and the science behind them. At the end of the book we'll cover how to find these mushrooms, as mushrooms or as supplements." ML

ISBN 978-1492854326

Table of Contents

What's behind 'Eating Mushrooms'?

There seems to always have been a significant amount of confusion on the safety of consuming mushrooms. There are a variety of mushrooms that are delicious if one were to pan sear them and include them to compliment a chicken marsala dish; however, there are also a spectrum of mushrooms that when used the wrong way become a dangerous poisonous substance. While mushrooms are exceptionally diverse in purpose, there is a way to distinguish each type of this fungus by shape, size, color, origin, and texture in order to tell each type of plant from one another. It is in the science of distinguishing each type of mushrooms that are edible that scientists and doctors have been able to develop many various benevolent substances that are used today in medical practice. In fact, some of the uses of the edible forms of this plant are even able to accomplish huge feats including, but not limited to, improving the immune system, fighting cancer, protect against HIV, reducing stress, and in some cases even fights against tuberculosis. These amazing qualities make the mushroom a huge benefit to both the scientific as well as medical realms.

Some of the mushrooms that are listed below can be found at your local supermarket, while other mushrooms are only found in exotic locations that have been documented through history. Through understanding the purpose of the intended use of various forms of mushrooms, one will be able to see a pattern form in the medical and scientific field of how particular medicines and chemicals originated. The study of mushrooms is a great way to build a foundation of understanding for specific types of medicines and chemicals that are believed to, and some proven to, alter the state of the body enough to produce positive physical results in the state of the health of the subject. Not all conclusions made about mushrooms have been extensively tested and theorized; however, there are tons of beliefs about the beneficial properties of mushrooms and their effect on the human body.

Nutritional mushrooms are one of the most promising and highest performing nutrition and 'curative' natural food source found to date. The challenge is, 'what mushrooms for what ailment'? That's the purpose of this direct, to the point, no fluff volume. This book was written for those interested in information on the following mushrooms, what they can do for you, and the science behind them. At the end of the book we'll cover how to find these mushrooms, as mushrooms or as supplements.

The Weird history of Edible Mushrooms

For a significant amount of time, edible mushrooms have always been considered one of the main sources of food for a majority of beings. Mushrooms have originated a concrete source of fuel for many living beings due to the ease in which one can obtain them naturally in the wild. Many mushrooms are present in grass, dirt, on the side of trees, etc. Therefore, many living beings would not see the challenge in relying on mushrooms as a main nutritional source. True, not all mushrooms are edible. In fact, some of them are so deadly that in the ancient times, they were often used as poisons against their enemies, knowing the targeted family would have its fair share of edible ones that do not only serve as a food source, but also plays a very important part in the field of medicine and nutrition. This way adding the poisonous mushrooms to the family's supply of mushrooms would be a seamless act and would go undetected.

According to the WHFoods, edible mushrooms such as maitake, button, shiitake and lobster have low fat and sodium. They are also rich in various vitamins and minerals that aids well in the nutrition and metabolism of the people who eat it. This is the reason for so many of these various mushrooms being included in dietary selections that are suggested by nutrition experts and health professional. If you study any of the premade meals that are offered by companies that claim that their premade meal offerings will aid in weight loss, there are almost always a number of choices with various types of mushrooms. This is so that the company can benefit from providing a good tasting and satisfying meal, and the customers can take advantage of the fact that there are metabolism-boosting properties in the mushrooms that are included in the dishes. Selected mushrooms meanwhile, are valued for their medical utility, a practice that has been with the human race since the Ayurvedic times more than 5000 years ago. Each different mushroom was distinguished through the look and feel of the mushroom, as well as the location in which the specific type of mushroom would grow. This way people would be able to note the reactions to the various types of mushrooms in order to be able to prescribe a specific mushroom for the ailment that the afflicted was facing. In fact, ancient Greeks call mushrooms "food of the gods" as they are known to help prevent diseases and strengthen the immune system. This would have been a common practice in those times because of the fact that the people looked to the gods for everything. The gods were considered to be in charge of every development in the lives of the people; therefore, if there were a naturally occurring food that was plentiful, easy to harvest, simple to locate, that had healing and physically beneficial properties, then this would have been considered to be a gift from the gods, as well as a food good enough for the gods. In the modern times, recent studies also show that certain species of mushrooms have the potential to be a preventive agent against HIV, other immune function disorders and cancer. Now that there have been so many advances in technology, science, and medicine, people are now able to draw more concrete conclusions about the benefits and uses of mushrooms. Society can use more than trial and error to figure out if a mushroom is edible or not, and what medical use it would be great for.

Agaricus Blazei

(Also known as Agaricus subrufescens, Agaricus brasiliensis and/or Agaricus rufotegulis) Commonly known as the hime-mitsutake mushrooms, these fungi are known to help strengthen the body's immune system and a preventive medical alternative against other diseases. Many people believe that by simply strengthening the body's natural immune system, one can be brought to the point of being able to fight off any disease that may develop in one's body. This is a common belief that is not necessarily tested or proven in any society with any concrete evidence. However, there have been enough people who have benefited greatly from the implementation of mushrooms like this one that they feel there is a trend with the results. Apart from these known and established properties, continuous studies are still being done on this mushroom as more and more useful discoveries and benefits are established and acknowledged by the scientific world.

A. blazei is popular in the Asian region in particular, including Korea, Taiwan and China for the claims that the said fungi is capable of preventing the proliferation of cancer cells, osteoporosis, diabetes, and a number of circulatory system disorders. It is interesting that the results that are found with each unique form of mushroom are proprietary to one system or one chain of parts that are all connected by function. There are also claims stating that the mushroom is capable of inducing calm that is able to help with relieving most patients from physical and emotional stress and disorders.

The presence of complex polysaccharides in the fungi is said to be the perpetrator of its anti-cancer capabilities. This is what makes the mushroom a valuable player in the quest for the cure for cancer. Other biochemical components, such as beta-glucans are said to inhibit the growth of the tumor and fully eliminate cancer cells. As claimed by scientists who conducted a rigorous study on this fungi in the laboratory and documented the various results by implementing these components of the mushroom in to the experiments as a controlled variable. The mushroom is also known to have antioxidant properties, and help effectively expel unwanted toxins in the body that potentially damages the tissues in the body. By removing the toxins from the body, the mushroom enables the body to have the time to heal from whatever negative elements were previously present.

As mentioned earlier, the A. blazei is also found to help prevent circulatory disorders such as high blood pressure and cholesterol, and helps dilate the blood vessels along the heart, making sure that there is enough space for the blood pumped to and from the heart to smoothly flow all over the different parts of the body. This is a vital discovery in the advantages to having mushrooms in the diet, science, and medicinal practices. As long as there are not any allergies with mushrooms present, then one would be able to greatly benefit from the power of mushrooms in regards to blood pressure and cholesterol. The medications that many doctors prescribe for blood pressure and cholesterol are typically riddled with side effects; by finding a homeopathic solution for the high blood pressure or bad cholesterol, one is not only protecting his or her body; however, he or she is also helping to heal his or her body without nasty side effects.

In recent studies, an extract from the mushroom A. blazei was gathered and analyzed in hopes to expand the medical and therapeutic capability of the species. By engaging with a plant in an isolated study of the reactions and changes due to the implementation of the fungus, scientists are able to make assumptions, and draw conclusions that eventually lead to hypotheses and hopefully proven theories. Scientists concluded that the fungi also showed anti-hypoallergenic, anti-arteriosclerosis, and anti-hypertriglyreidemic properties, making it a very useful source of food and nutrition. This study proved that this type of mushroom would be great to use in the common household during various times of the year. Many people all over the world suffer from allergies, and if including a mushroom in the diet of a person could help to fight against the painful symptoms of the allergy suffering public, then it could be assumed that many people, barring those who are allergic, would be interested in participating.

Agarikon

Usually found along the tree barks in various forests worldwide, this mushroom has penetrated through the nutrition and health industry for thousands of years already. In ancient times, the Greeks called Agarikon the "elixir of life", as it showcases several medical capabilities that are valued by many. In North America on the other hand, the Agarikon is commonly called the "tree biscuits" or "bread of ghosts" for their appearance, and a traditional belief that this fungi holds spiritual powers often used by Shamans to cure ailments allegedly caused by the supernatural forces. In a variety of different cultures, mushrooms were used to ward of negative presences, or on the other side to bring positivity to one's life. It can be assumed that due to the patterns of positive effects that mushrooms had on the physical body of the humans, that they then assumed that the plant also had other supernatural powers. Remember, there was not always a scientific process to back up the medicinal belief systems of a society. Therefore, if a mushroom healed a person's affliction, then it was believed to be an act of the gods or supernatural in and of itself in some way. Consequently, the power of the mushroom would be considered that the plant should be lumped in with other supernatural occurrences.

Some of the mushrooms in the Agarikon family can cause a modest or mild psychedelic experience, (another reason why supernatural powers and religions aspects have been attributed to them). It is for this reason that it is recommended to you to acquire a good quality supplement with the benefits of Agarikon mushrooms contained, rather than to pick your own, or purchase these mushrooms, (although it can be done). Those that produce a psychedelic experience are generally illegal in any event, and are much more expensive than just getting a high quality supplement. There is no danger of psychedelic reactions from an Agarikon based supplement and these supplements deliver tremendous anti-inflammatory benefits.

Agarikon mushrooms generally work as an anti-inflammatory and antibacterial agent. These are amazing benefits to the human body and for our health, (both in healing and maintaining). There are many largely common conditions that are affected by the presence of an anti-inflammatory, or an antibacterial substance. Scientific tests were conducted and it was, in fact, shown that this fungi actively reacts against certain viruses including, but not limited to, the bird flu, the swine flu, herpes, and cowpox viruses. Further, it was confirmed by the Institute for Tuberculosis Research in Illinois, Chicago show that this edible mushroom potentially shows activity against tuberculosis. This suggests that the fungi may also be a useful anti-tuberculosis agent and may help the medical experts find better ways to cure the disease that has been pestering the human race ever since before the 1500's.

Agarikon is widely used as an effective natural health supplement, helping improve the body, the circulatory system and immune system as a whole. Scientists explain that this fungi is capable of preventing cardiac arrests, lowering the cholesterol level of the patients, and preventing and controlling diabetes. The circulatory system is a major player in the highly efficient and effective operation of the human body. As soon as the circulatory system is negatively affected or restricted, then the condition of the body begins to deteriorate. Cholesterol and diabetes are two factors that can negatively affect the circulatory system, and are affected by the circulatory system, they go hand in hand with one another. Therefore, if implementing the Agarikon mushroom is able to positively affect the circulatory system, then this is how it would be able to positively affect the presence of processing of cholesterol, and controlling of diabetes.

Black Trumpet

(Scientific name: Craterellus cornucopioides also known as 'the horn of plenty', as well as the black chanterelle, or in French 'trompette de la mort' which means 'trumpet of the dead' – ironic due to its wonderful antibacterial properties)

This thin, black fungi initially looks so unappealing that you would either think it looks poisonous or end up not noticing it at all. In reality however, this mushroom plays a very important role in the culinary industry. This mushroom, often ignored or feared, is actually a very yummy ingredient that ensures the unique taste of mushroom in various dishes. There are many dishes in Asian cuisine that utilize the black trumpet mushroom as an exotic and unique ingredient that sets the flavors of the cuisine apart from others all around the world. This type of mushroom has a distinct taste and texture that will be appealing to some and not others. However, the point is that it is edible and can complement some dishes with an extraordinarily different and seldom used flavor.

Apart from the culinary prowess of this mushroom, traditional medicine practitioners also use the black trumpet as an efficient natural medicine to cure a number of diseases and ailments. Like many other forms of mushrooms, the black trumpet also possesses a variety of natural beneficial elements that are believed to help improve the processes of the human body. As in the rest of the edible mushrooms, this fungi has a lot of antibacterial and antioxidant properties, making this simple looking mushroom into a delicious and healthy ingredient. The antibacterial properties will help people to fight off many varieties of diseases before they can develop in to something much worse, while the antioxidant properties help in a number of ways. Antioxidants are used in the body for a spectrum of reasons; some antioxidants help to reduce stress, and others fight free radicals that are potentially harmful to the health of the person affected by the free radicals.

While some consumers remain in the dark about the advantages to including this fungus in his or her diet, other consumers frequently include this fungus in his or her daily life. These people claim that the edible mushroom may also be a good health supplement against asthma and muscle pain. Many people around the world suffer from frequent muscle pain and asthma, and therefore are always looking for a new way to battle against these conditions. By including mushrooms in his or her daily live, a number of people have found that mushrooms help to reduce the amount of suffering from muscle pain and asthma. People who are suffering from obesity also prefer adding the black trumpet to their menu. The biochemical components of this mushroom actually helps enhance the metabolic activity in the body, effectively helping the obese lose their weight efficiently. It is easier to add a delicious component to a meal in order to lose weight instead of switching to eating only cardboard-like energy bars. This mushroom helps to make weight loss an attainable goal for those who struggle with obesity or excess weight on a regular basis.

Turkey Tail

(Also called Coriolus versicolor as well as Polyporus versicolor) Popularly known for being a visually appealing mushroom, the Turkey Tail, scientifically named as Trametes versicolor, proves that it is not just a good looking fungi, but one with great function and value in the scientific and medical world as well. Popularly used as a medicinal herb, this fungi is known as Kawaratake in Japan, meaning cloud mushroom and is used as a medical supplement in China, commonly called as the Yun Zhi. It usually grows in colonies and more often found in the Pacific Northwest of the world, growing from May to December. Therefore, it is harvested during this time and used for its beneficial properties all over the world.

One of Turkey Tails popular biochemical components is the Polysaccharide-K (PSK). This is the main component of an anticancer drug approved in Japan, which is Krestin. Krestin is generally composed of extracted PSK from the Turkey Tail, and is a known anticancer agent. Many mushrooms are believed to be able to help eliminate cancer cells, however, this mushroom has been tested extensively in order to find the exact benefits and components that might help to fight cancer. In fact, the scientific world has embraced the fungi's potential as an anticancer agent, with United States' FDA subsequently approving the project of subjecting human patients to undergo trials for using the Turkey Tail as an anticancer agent in 2012. This is a huge step for the consideration of the advantages of the elements present in mushrooms to be thought of as a great combatant for cancer. Many people, all over the world, struggle with the battle with cancer, if the answer to beating cancer could be in something as simple as mushrooms, then that could be a beautiful discovery. Being that mushrooms are so plentiful and easy to grow or harvest, the answer could be in great supply someday soon.

Turkey Tail is also famous for the Polysaccharide-P (PSP), which is found to be a good antiviral agent. This allows scientists to view the fungi's potential as it could inhibit the proliferation of HIV virus in the body. It is because of the fact that HIV is a virus that the antivirus agents that are potentially present in the turkey tail mushrooms could help to be the answer to fighting the spread and effects of HIV. This, in effect, helps strengthen and boost the body's immune system from possible viral and bacterial attacks.

Apart from the scientifically founded research on this mushroom's effectiveness, Turkey Tail is also known to be a therapeutic and medical supplement for a number of diseases and ailments. This fungi, is in fact being used in the traditional Chinese medicine for centuries now to help heal pulmonary disorders such as reducing phlegm and clearing the dampness, increase a person's energy, and boosting the body's defense system from acquiring chronic diseases. Turkey Tail is also used for reducing the inflammation in the body, particularly in the urinary, respiratory and digestive tracts. Further, Turkey Tail is also known to help improve a patient's body and become a medical supplement against liver ailments such as hepatitis. The liver is the organ in the body that helps to filter out and process toxins; by including this mushroom in the regular diet of an individual, it is believed that the liver functions can be improved to the

point that the body is functioning more efficiently and effectively. Therefore, preparing the human body to fight
off chronic diseases and predisposed diseases in order
to reach a healthier state of living.

Cordyceps

Cordyceps is also a truly important mushroom for your health. Like the other edible mushrooms, this fungi is part of an ancient practice in the Tibetan and Chinese traditional medicine. Despite its prominent characteristics as a fungus, Cordyceps is well known to provide health and therapeutic benefits especially to the respiratory and circulatory system. Therefore, resulting in better oxygenation of the muscular systems, alertness, and brain functions. It can consequently be hypothesized that extended exposure to this type of mushroom could result in a significant improvement in overall health and overall body functions.

Cordyceps is prominently used in traditional medicine in the Asian region. In fact, Chinese Traditional Medicine has been using this mushroom as a medical supplement for various ailments for about 300 years already. The fungi used to be abundant, but restriction of habitat and over exploration restricted the mushroom's proliferation and in effect, severely decreased the species' number. Nevertheless, the fungi is duly cultured along the forest lands of China and continues to provide the science world with its usefulness. It is a painful situation to discover that a previously plentiful plant now regarded as a medicinal component with so many excellent advantages is now in restricted supply.

Cordyceps is used in the field of traditional medicine for many purposes and treatment of several ailments, including antioxidant, stress resistance, strengthening and immune booster, and anti-ageing. It has biochemical components which help stimulate the immune system, helping it protect the body from any possible viral or bacterial infection. The presence of cytokines in Cordyceps also contributes in the prevention of inflammation in the body. The combination of an anti-inflammatory and an anti-viral element to this one type of mushroom make it a strong competitor for medical use. Many viruses develop into infections because of the inflammation that they cause in the various sinus cavities of the body. However, if you fight the virus and prevent the inflammation in the first place then one would be in a better place to not ever suffer from an infection caused by that virus.

In traditional Chinese Medicine, this fungus is commonly used as a medical supplement in treating kidney diseases by protecting the organ from deteriorating. The kidneys are an exceedingly important part of the body and how it functions. Therefore, protecting the kidneys at all costs is imperative to the proper functioning of the human body. By taking proactive measures, one would be able to protect the kidneys from deteriorating and result in overall improved health. It is also commonly used as treatment for respiratory problems including asthma, shortness of breath, and coughing.

Recent scientific studies meanwhile, focus on discovering more properties of Cordyceps and figuring out its effectiveness in inhibiting the growth of cancer cells among patients. As of present, the mushroom is considered a medical supplement as it helps restore the production of white blood cells after cancer treatments such as radiation and chemotherapy. This could also be in conjunction with the preservation of the kidneys as the kidneys are a filtering system in the body. Frequently, when mushrooms are found to have cancer fighting properties it is also combined with an element of the mushroom that also helps to improve the efficiency of the organs that filter toxins out of the body like the liver and kidneys.

Lion's Mane

(Well known as the Lion's Mane Mushroom, or Bearded Tooth Mushroom, sometimes the Hedgehog Mushroom, even Satyr's Beard, ask well as the Bearded Hedgehog Mushroom, pom pom mushroom, and the Bearded Tooth Fungus) The Lion's Mane, is named Hericium erinaceus in the scientific world, and is one of the most well-known traditional Chinese medicine ingredients. This mushroom, famous for its biochemical component called the NGF or the Nerve Growth Factor, is fully recommended in the scientific world for being able to help treat some of the most difficult health problems. In fact, as it is a very prestigious herb, the Lion's Mane was considered rare in the ancient Chinese times and only the emperors were privileged to eat them.

The presence of the polypeptides and fatty acids are said to be the proponents of this mushroom's effective healing capabilities. Research and scientific studies show that enzymes and other components such as oleanolic acids, polysaccharides, and adenosine are some factors that helps modulate and boost the immune system. It also helps enhance the digestive process and provide anti-inflammatory effects.

This fungi also helps in the effective functioning of the circulatory system as it helps regulate blood pressure and cholesterol. The presence of NGF on the other hand, allows the Lion's Mane to effectively battle against neurological disorders such as dementia, Alzheimer's disease and other peripheral neurological dysfunctions.

Current scientific studies now show that Lion's Mane may, like its fellow edible mushroom families, have the potential to protect the body against the proliferation of cancer cells. In a 2011 study, it was found that this fungi helps fight leukemia. The same year, an extensive study also showed the plant's potential as an anti-cancer agent when the cancer cells successfully reduced its size after introducing the plant extract. This goes to show that the plant may indeed have an effective and promising contribution against cancer.

Maitake

(Also called Hen-of-the-woods, Signorina, Ram's head and the Sheep's head) The Maitake mushroom or Grifola frondosa is a large, fan shaped mushroom that is usually found along fallen bee or beech tree trunks. This mushroom proved its worth to the civilization not only as a rich source of food for daily consumption, but also as a helpful traditional medicine. In fact, various scientific research from scientists in Asia in particular, presents a very huge number of ailments this mushroom has the potential of either curing or preventing.

One of the main components of Maitake is the huge presence of high-molecular-weight of polysaccharides, which helps in maintaining the blood pressure and cholesterol levels, boost the immune system, become a useful anti-ageing and anti-inflammatory agents, and treat heavier ailments including cancer, hemorrhoids, and potential anti-cancer activities.

The presence of the polysaccharide known as the beta-glucan provides for the antitumor properties of Maitake, helping kill malignant tumors and cells in the body. Further studies on beta-glucan extracted from Maitake are currently being assessed to test for its effectiveness on patients with relapse or those with cancer in a progressive phase.

Maitake is also known to have antioxidant properties which help cleanse the body from toxins and reduce oxidative damages. The presence of fibrous nutrients and components in the mushroom also makes it a good agent for weight loss. Antioxidants will assist in weight loss by helping the body to fight free radicals, and flush out the unwanted fats and oils from the body.

Oyster Mushroom

(Can also go by the name of Abalone mushroom, or Tree mushroom) Oyster mushrooms have been part of the traditional medicine. It has played an important part both in the field of medicine and dining, as most cuisines, especially those from Eastern and East Asia, use this mushroom as an integral part of their dishes. Majority found in China, the oyster mushroom has been used in the country as a therapeutic supplement and is commonly called "medical mushrooms".

Oyster Mushrooms are known as good antioxidant and antibacterial agents. This mushroom is rich in minerals and vitamins including phosphorus, vitamins B1, B2 and C, niacin, folic acid, calcium and iron. They also have potassium which helps prevent heart disease and regulate blood pressure. This is consequently a great source of boosting one's metabolism and immune system thanks to the various elements that improve the body's overall health.

The edible fungi is known to have a biochemical compound called the ergothioneine, which is known to protect the cells and build up immunity in the body. This biochemical component is responsible for the mushroom's antioxidant properties. It also contains vitamin D, which helps strengthen the bones.

Oyster mushrooms are known to be effective therapeutic supplements aimed to help boost and protect the body from ailment such as Hepatitis, constipation, hyperacidity and anemia.

Recent studies also show that Oyster Mushrooms may actually contribute to the prevention of cancerous cell proliferation in the body. As of present, cancer research is concentrated on the edible mushrooms as a whole and investigations on their capability as a probable factor in defeating cancer is looked at.

Poria cocos

Known as Fu-Ling in Chinese, Poria cocos is one of the widely accepted and often used ingredient as a therapeutic supplement in China's traditional herbal medicine. Mainly used as a sedative, this mushroom is well recognized for its good potential as an alternative medicine and is currently looked at by most research scientists to magnify the list of its benefits to human beings.

Poria cocos is currently looked at as a possible supplement for prevention of cancer due to the presence of monosaccharides, which is known for its anti-tumor properties. This mushroom also helps prevent inflammation and contributes in the treatment of joint pains and against rheumatoid arthritis.

The presence of Triterpenes on the other hand, enhances the fungi's capability as an anti-diabetic property as it helps regulate blood sugar level and boosts the insulin action and production in the body.

Poria cocos. (Also known as Wolfiporia extensa sclerotium, hoelen, tuckahoe, poria, China root, matsuhodo, and fu ling). This healthy mushroom is rich in organic acids such as tumulosic acid and pachymic acid, effectively giving a tranquilizing and diuretic effect. Apart from being a sedative for its tranquilizing effect, this mushroom is also commonly used in Chinese traditional herbal medicine as a preventive medicine against dizziness, nervousness, urination, diarrhea, kidney health, Edema, and Chronic Fatigue.

Reishi

(Also called the lingzhi mushroom and is often associated with Ganoderma lucidum and Ganoderma tsugae, as it's very closely related). Reishi is one of the edible mushrooms that has been a part of the traditional herbal medicine in Eastern Asia for centuries. Unlike other edible mushrooms however, Reishi is more known for its therapeutic and pharmaceutical contribution rather than its nutritional value.

Reishi, unlike other mushrooms, is known to have two active major components; the triterpenes and the polysaccharides. These are believed to be the main proponents in the fungi's pharmaceutical capability, including its antibacterial and anticancer properties. Within the spores of the mushroom are also several long-chained fatty acids, which provides the fungi's antitumor capabilities.

Reishi is known to help boost the immune system. It is often promoted as an immuno-modulating agent due to its capability to improve the body's resistance against bacterial and viral infection, and the removal of malignant cells. It is also a good antioxidant agent, which helps decrease the risk of cell mutation and damages.

The presence of polysaccharides, particularly the ganoderans A and B, also makes this mushroom a good anti-diabetes agent. These polysaccharides also help increase plasma insulin and decrease the hepatic glycogen content in the body, strengthening the body's excretory system as a whole.

The presence of peptidoglycan in Reishi also allows the mushroom to have hypotensive and hypertensive properties, contributing to the effective stabilization of the blood pressure and cholesterol levels. The mushroom fungi also have dietary fibers, making it a good dietary supplement to support the health of its consumers.

Shiitake

(Also known as the Sawtooth oak mushroom, or the black forest mushroom, or just black mushroom, but sometimes known as the golden oak mushroom or the oakwood mushroom. In the past this mushroom species was known as Lentinus edodes or Agaricus edodes). For more than 6,000 years, Shiitake has been a part of the traditional herbal medicine in the Chinese and the rest of Eastern Asia Region. The nutritional and pharmaceutical value of Shiitake is, in fact, so well received that it has become a symbolic figure of longevity and good life. Even now, the usefulness of this mushroom has expanded and is widely appreciated by thousands all over the world.

Shiitake mushrooms commonly grow in the forests in Asia. It is, in fact, considered second to the most cultivated edible mushrooms in the world due to its nutritional and pharmaceutical properties. It contains a lot of polysaccharides, fatty acids, nutrients and vitamins that provides effective therapeutic properties to its consumers. In fact, most nutrition experts find the presence of these nutrients just as important and worthy to put shiitake mushrooms as part of a balanced diet.

Shiitake mushroom promotes a lot of health benefits, most of which are proven and supported by several clinical studies. One of the key findings in Shiitake mushroom's health benefits is its antitumor property due to the presence of a fascinating polypeptide named lentinan. The lentinan found on shiitake mushrooms help hinder the development and proliferation of cancer cells in the body. A recent study also shows that the fungi is also an effective agent to prevent tooth decay.

The mushroom is also rich in protein, vitamins, potassium, vitamin B and copper. These effectively promote the cardiovascular benefits of the mushroom into the body. This in turn, also helps regulate the blood pressure and cholesterol in the body by reducing the production of immune cell adhesion molecules that causes plaques in the arteries. By reducing the presence of the amount of plaques in the arteries, and improving blood pressure and the processing of cholesterol, one can conclude that this type of mushroom helps to fight against heart disease. This is a great development in the world of using mushrooms as medicine, because a significant amount of the world's population suffers from different aspects of heart disease every single year. Therefore, it is imperative that society finds all the various ways to reduce the risk of heart disease in the world as a whole.

Like other edible mushrooms, shiitake mushroom also has an antioxidant property due to the presence of key minerals such as zinc, selenium and manganese. The presence of ergothioneine in the mushroom also plays a key role in the production of energy for the mitochondria, strengthening the heart's health and the entire circulatory system.

Fight cancer, HIV, and tuberculosis and much more

There are many various types of mushrooms that are easily available to the general public at a local food store; however, there are other mushrooms that are more challenging to obtain than others. Some mushrooms have been regarded as possessing medical healing and preventative elements for thousands of years. While other mushrooms are recently being discovered as having advantages to the immune system, or even cancer fighting properties. There are a variety of commonalities that thread the benefits of most mushrooms together. However, there are also differences between the major advantages to each unique species of mushroom. You can distinguish between various types of mushrooms through the observation of their size, shape, color, texture, and the location in which they originated. This is the way that many cultures throughout history have distinguished which mushroom is believed to help with what ailment. Now there are scientific and medical studies that help the public to understand the various uses and properties that each type of mushroom has. Now that science has the ability to test, and document the reactions and changes that are present after the implementation of specific mushrooms into one's diet, maybe they will be able to find a concrete way for mushrooms to be used to fight larger obstacles like cancer, HIV, and tuberculosis.

How can I get the benefits of these mushrooms if I am not someone who is able to shop for them, of find them growing wild?

We are very fortunate today to have reputable supplement companies that can provide the active nutritional components of these mushrooms. You can also find some of them for sale in farmers markets and as a specialty tea in Asian stores. If you find a supplement, one way to see if it is quality is to make a note if it is an NSF GMP manufacture. NSF means International/Good Manufacturing Practices, and such manufacturing plants are inspected and tested, as well as the raw ingredients, so that consumers can be assured that they are getting what is stated on the label. Of course, there are non-GMP production facilities that are very high quality as well, and good companies that choose to not get certified as an NSF GMP product. For example a great many businesses are not members of the BBB (Better Business Bureau) but are very reputable firms.

Bottom line: you get what you pay for, and with the Internet you can look for most products to see what others say about them. The key point is to start using these amazing healing mushrooms now with some quality brand. You can experiment with different brands as you learn more about them. Mushroom supplements are a lot less expensive than health care costs! To your health!